The Purpose of this Book

Every year tens of thousands of people including doctors, medical students, paramedics, nurses, nursing students, and others involved in the care and treatment of cardiac patients, get introduced to echocardiography; aka Echo or Ultrasound of the Heart.

The principles of echo are founded in physics although the interpretation of the results, e.g. color flow echo, shows that the use of Doppler shift and the direction of blood flow was not fully appreciated by those developing Cardiac Echo. In physics Doppler shift is the result of an object traveling away from the observer. As a result, the wavelength increases and the color shifts towards red. Objects traveling towards you compress the wavelength and the color shift is towards violet. In the world of Echocardiography, physicians flipped this scenario and red is blood flowing towards the transducer placed on the chest.

Thus in physics red is away from the observer, while in Cardiology red is toward the observer. This fundamental error was corrected when Transesophageal Echo (TEE) was developed. For this book we will focus on Transthoracic Echo (TTE) – or conventional[1] echo.

Nonetheless, the principles remain the same and this book will provide you with the basic information you need to know, to understand Cardiac Echo.

---

[1] Conventional changes with time. Color flow echocardiography was only being introduced into Cardiology when I was a Cardiology Fellow.

Understanding Basic Echocardiography.

By: Dr. Richard M. Fleming
Physicist – Nuclear Cardiologist

Non-Invasive Cardiology

- Echocardiography
    - Utilizing sound waves to obtain images of the heart
    - 2D, M-mode and Color Flow Doppler Echocardiography
- Myocardial Perfusion Imaging
    - Using nuclear isotopes to obtain images of the heart
    - Planar
    - SPECT (single photon emission computed tomography)
    - PET (positron emission tomography)

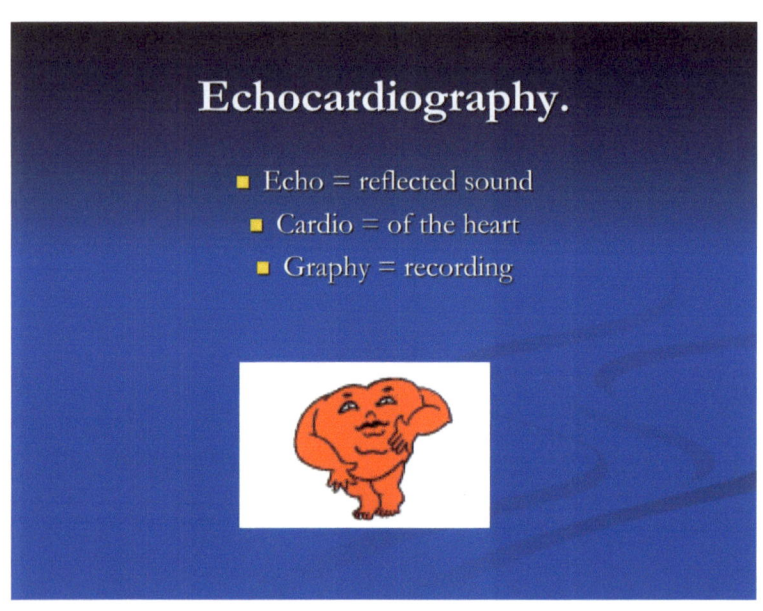

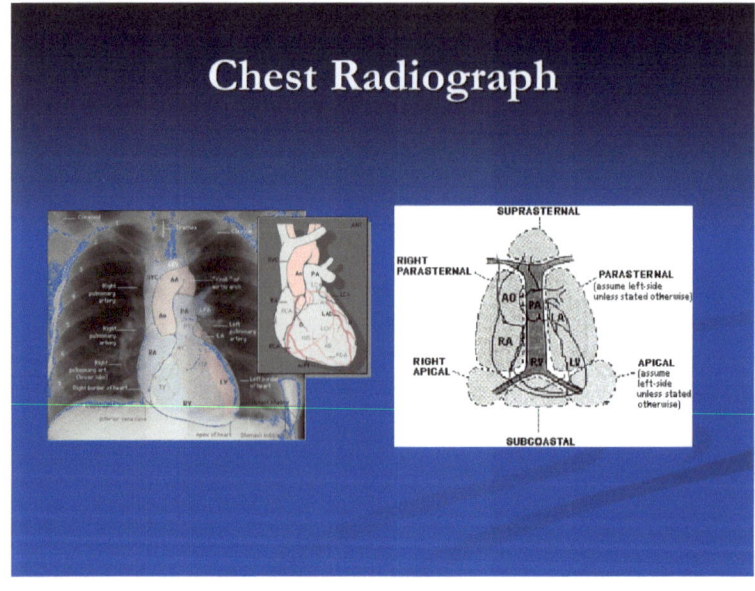

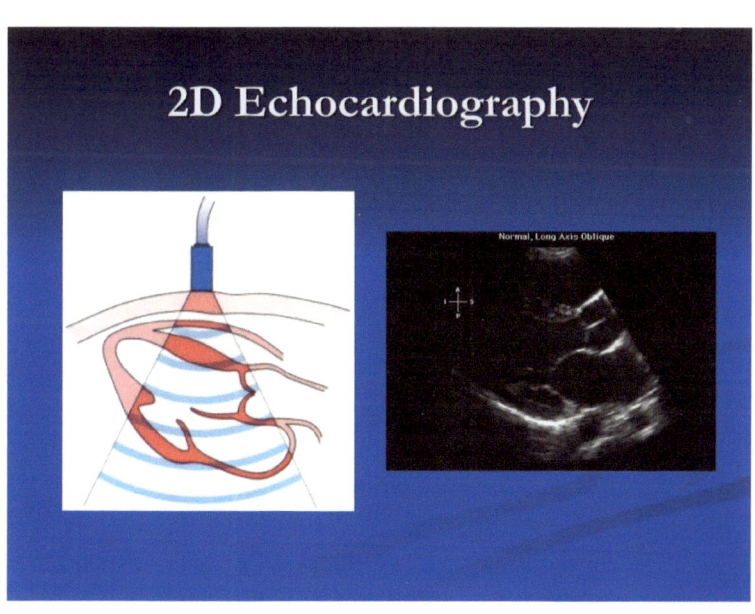

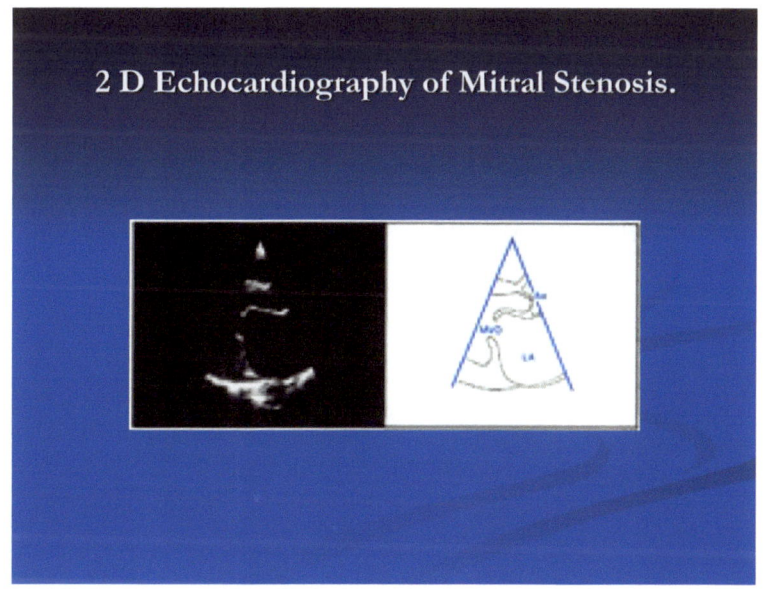

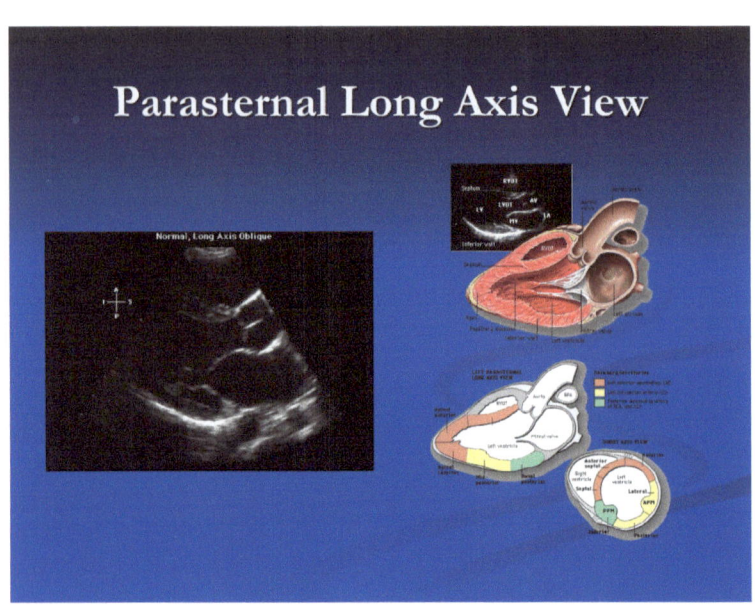
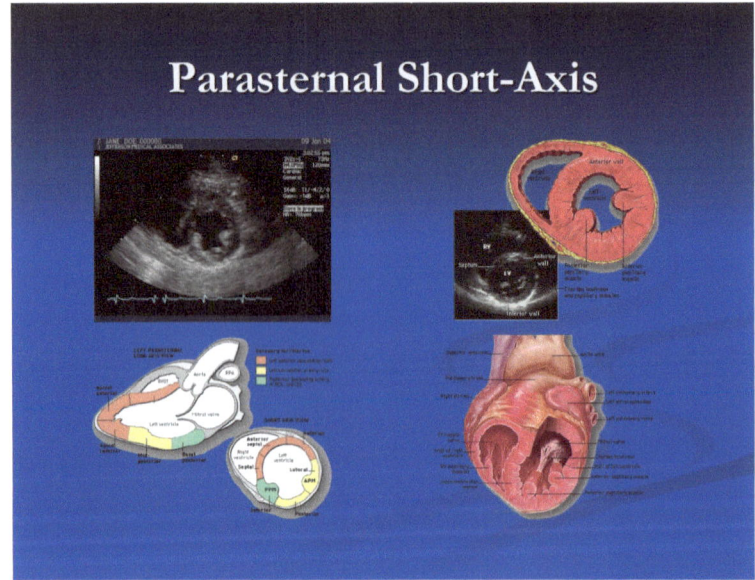

Short Axis View

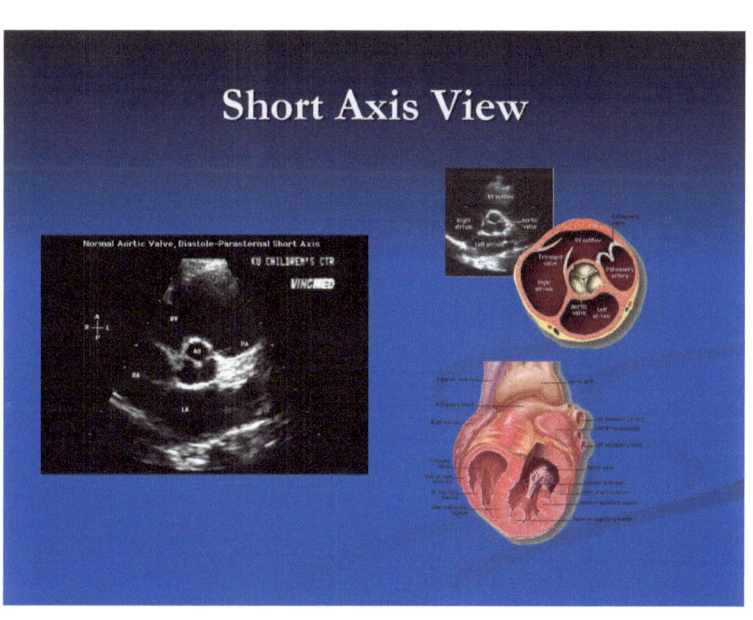

Apical 4 Chamber View

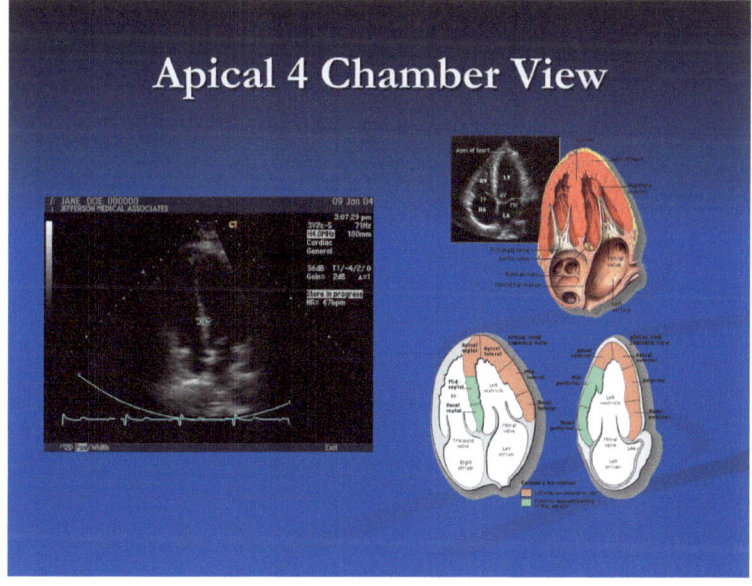

Apical 2 Chamber View

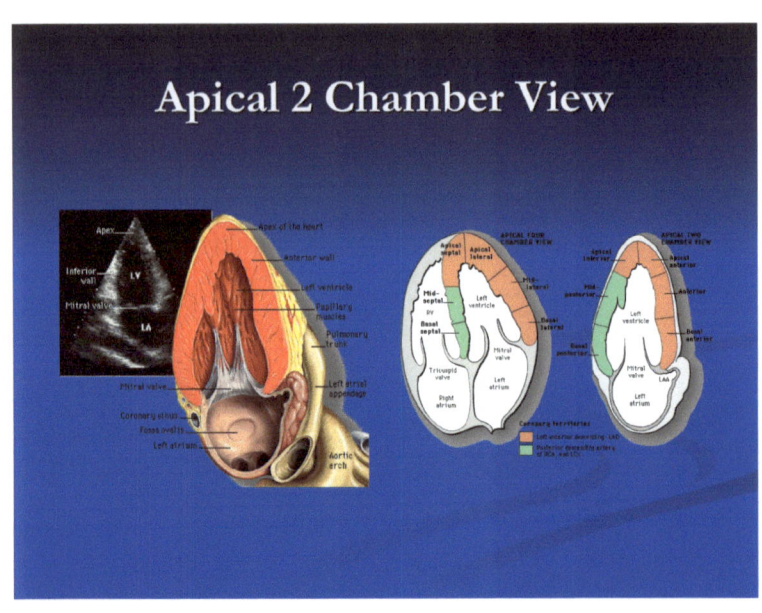

Suprasternal Notch

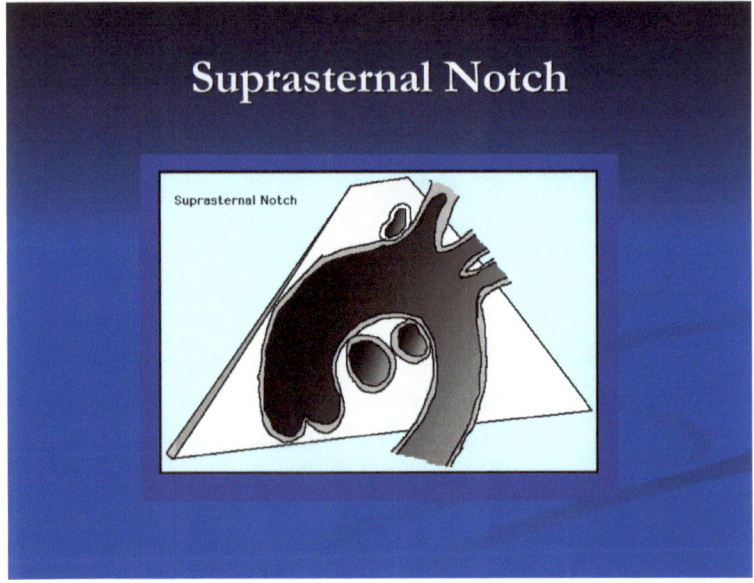

Sub-xyphoid View

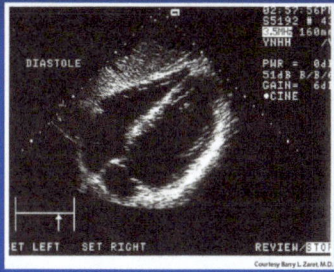
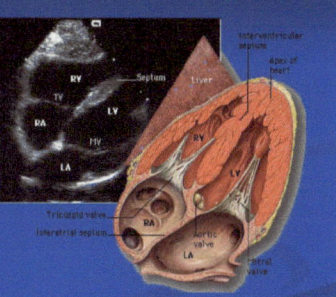

Subcostal View
IVC, Eustachian Valve & RA pressures.

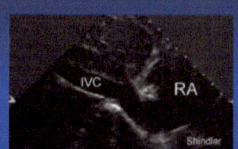

- RA pressures (inhalation or sniff)
  - IVC collapse = 5 mm Hg
  - Partial IVC collapse = 14 mm Hg
  - Non-reactive (no collapse) = 20 mm Hg

2 D & M-mode Together.

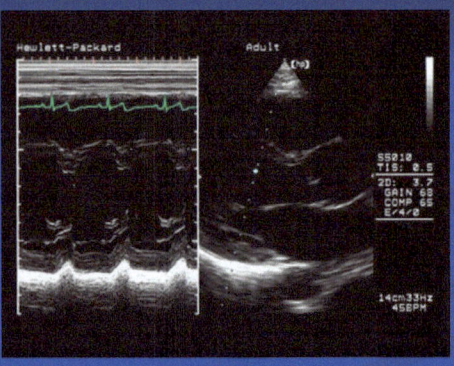

M-mode Echocardiography.
Measurements.

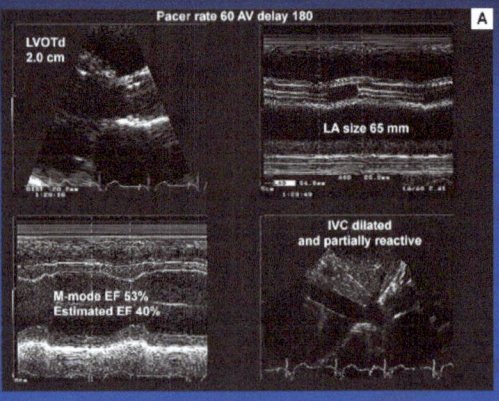

TR leads to RV overload (enlarged RV) and paradoxical motion of Septum.

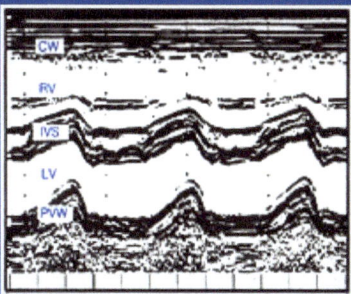

LVEF from M-mode of LV

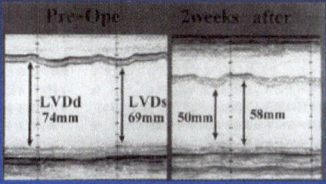

- LVEF from M-mode
  - LVFS* = LVEDD - LVESD/LVEDD
    - LVFS = (74-69/74) = 0.067
      - LVEF = (LVFS x 1.7)(100) = 11.5%
  - LVFS = LVEDD – LVESD/LVEDD
    - LVFS = (58-50/58) = 0.138
      - LVEF = (LVFS x 1.7)(100) = 23.4%
- These two studies show the before and after effect of CHF treatment.

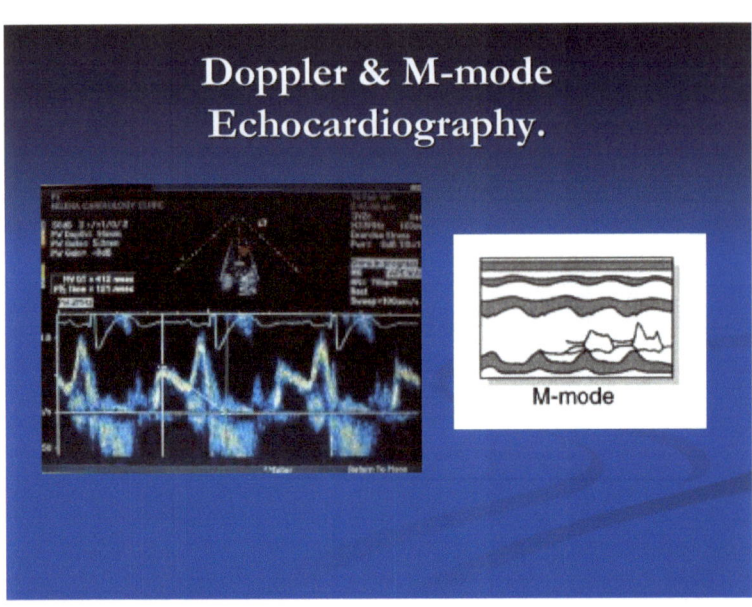

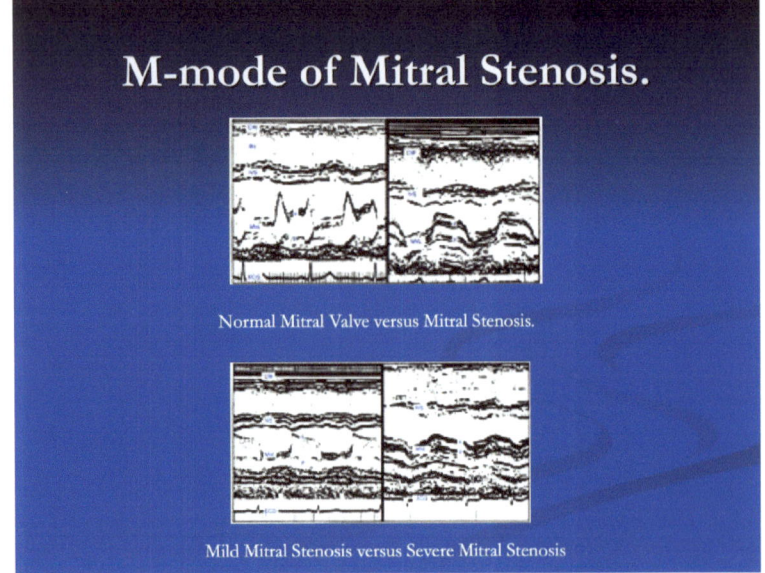

Mitral and Tricuspid Stenosis Secondary to RHD.

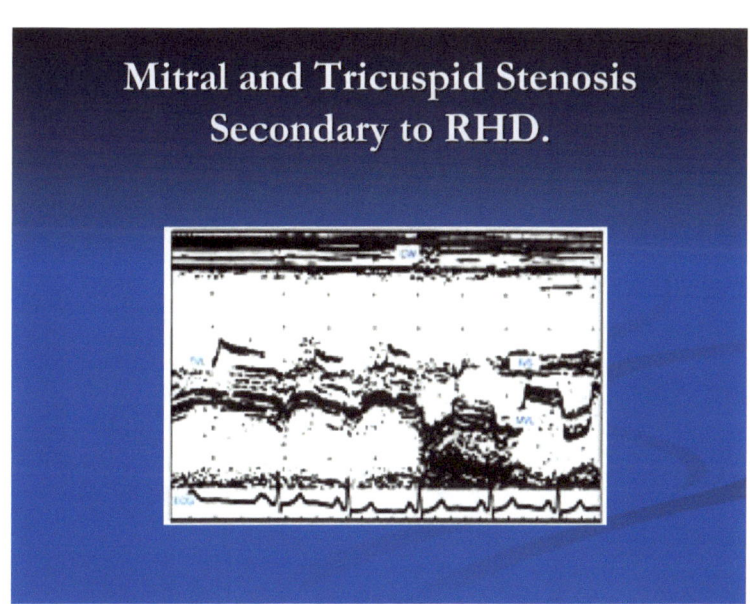

M-mode Evaluation of LV Wall Thickness - Apical 4 and 2 Chamber Views.

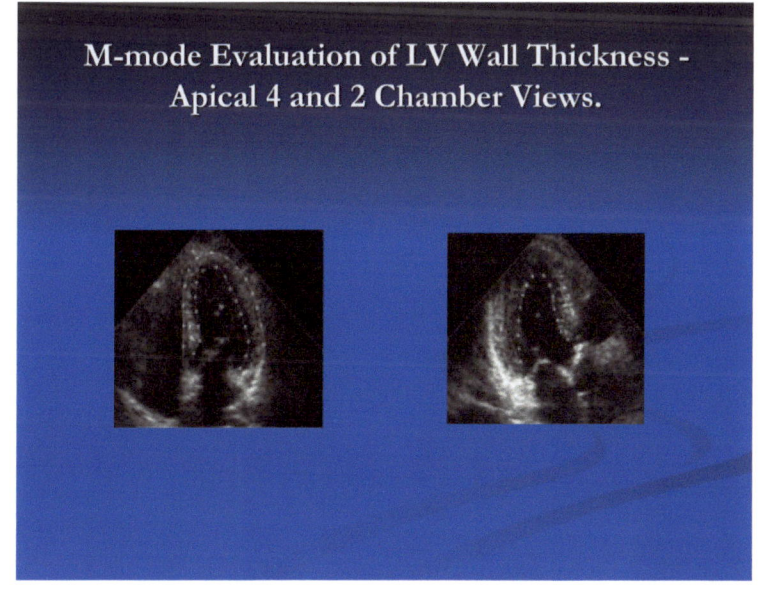

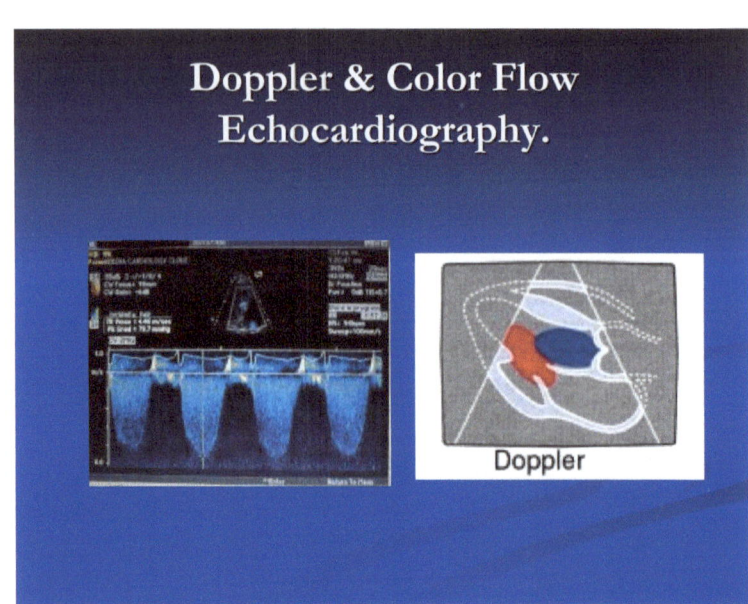

Doppler & Color Flow Echocardiography.

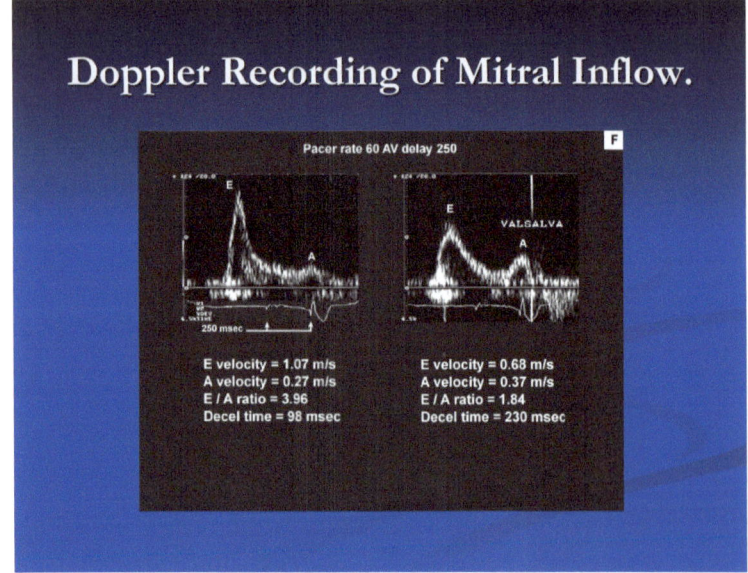

Doppler Recording of Mitral Inflow.

E velocity = 1.07 m/s
A velocity = 0.27 m/s
E / A ratio = 3.96
Decel time = 98 msec

E velocity = 0.68 m/s
A velocity = 0.37 m/s
E / A ratio = 1.84
Decel time = 230 msec

2 Dimensional (2 D) Echocardiography with Doppler.

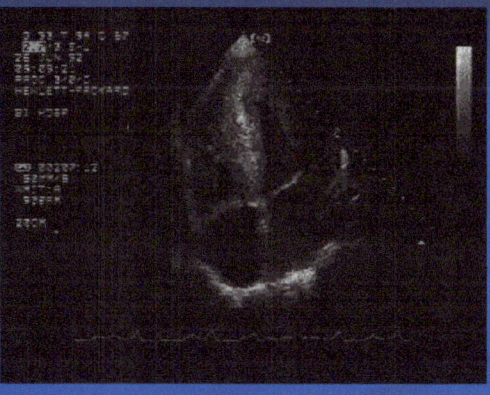

Tricuspid Regurgitation.

Tricuspid Regurgitation. Ventricularization of RA Pressures.

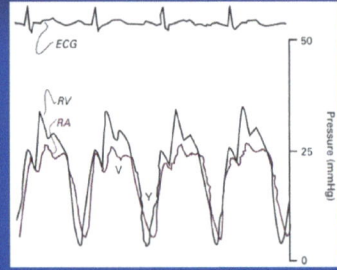

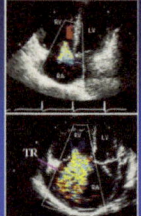

ECHO Assessment of PAH

Based on presence of Tricuspid Regurgitation

Using Doppler and Pressure Gradients to Determine Cardiac Pressures, Valve Areas & Shunts.

- TR can be used to calculate RVSP
- PR can be used to calculate (Pulmonary Pressures)
  - MPAP using Peak Pressure
  - End diastolic pressure
- RVOT of pulmonary flow = 79 – (0.45 x AC)
  - MPAP using acceleration time.
  - The shorter the AC, the greater the pulmonary pressures.
- When a VSD is present.
  - VSD gradient
  - RVSP = LVSP – VSD pressure.
- LV(E)SP = sBP + AoV gradient

Bernoulli (Pressure Gradient) Equation.

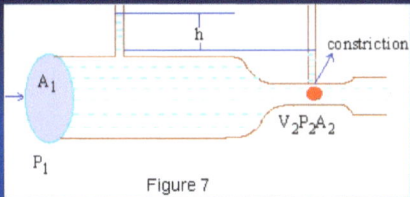

Figure 7

- Pressure Gradients occur across narrowing.
- Pressure = $4(V_2^2 - V_1^2)$
- Assuming V1 < 1.0 m/s
- Then Pressure = $4(V_2)^2$

Using PR and TR to Determine RV and PAP pressures.

- If you have PR (top)
  - Mean PAP =
    - Peak PR $V^2 \times 4 = X$ mmHg
    - eg. $(3^2 \times 4) = 36$ mm Hg
  - End diastolic PR pressure = (EDV^2) x 4 + RA pressure (sniff test).
    - Eg. $(1.3^2) \times 4 = 6.76$ (~7) + RA pressure (partial collapse = 10), so 7 + 10 = 17 mm Hg.
- If you don't have PR, but have TR, then you can only calculate RVSP
  - RVSP = $4V^2$ + Rap
  - RVSP = $4(2.7^2)$ + 10 = 39 mm Hg

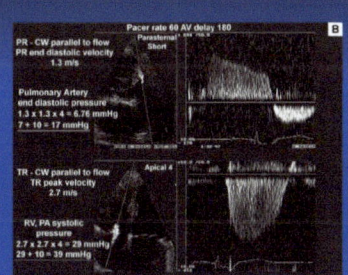

Right heart pressures (Pulm HTN)
Normal = 18-25 mm Hg
Mild HTN = 30-40 mm Hg
Moderate HTN = 40-70 mm Hg
Severe HTN = > 70 mm Hg

Transesophageal Approach to RVOT to Look at Pulmonary Valve & Flow.

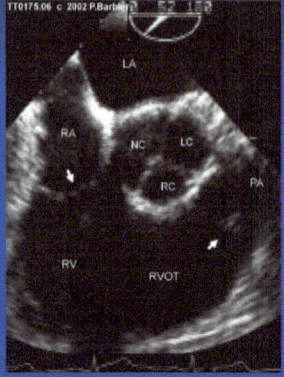
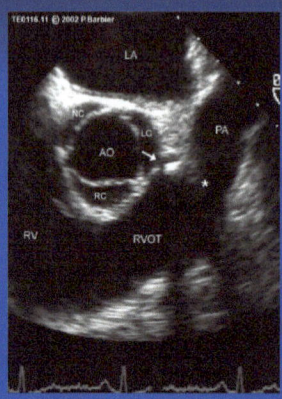

Using Pulmonary Doppler of RVOT to Determine MPAP from Forward Flow through Pulmonary Valve.

- Mean PAP can be determined by both
  - peak PR velocity or
  - Using parasternal long axis to measure acceleration time of pulmonary flow through RVOT.
- Acceleration time (AC) is time to peak velocity.
  - The shorter the AC the greater the pulmonary pressure (PHTN).
- MPAP = 79 – (0.45 x AC)
  - If AC is 130 msec, then
    - MPAP = 79 – (0.45x130) = 20 mm Hg [Normal Pulm Pressure]
  - If AC is 50 msec, then
    - MPAP = 79 – (0.45x50) = 57 mm Hg [Pulm HTN]

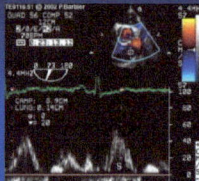
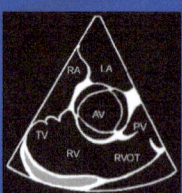

Unlike using PR or TR for pressures,
If MPAP is > 40 mm Hg = Severe PHTN.

Pulmonary Stenosis.

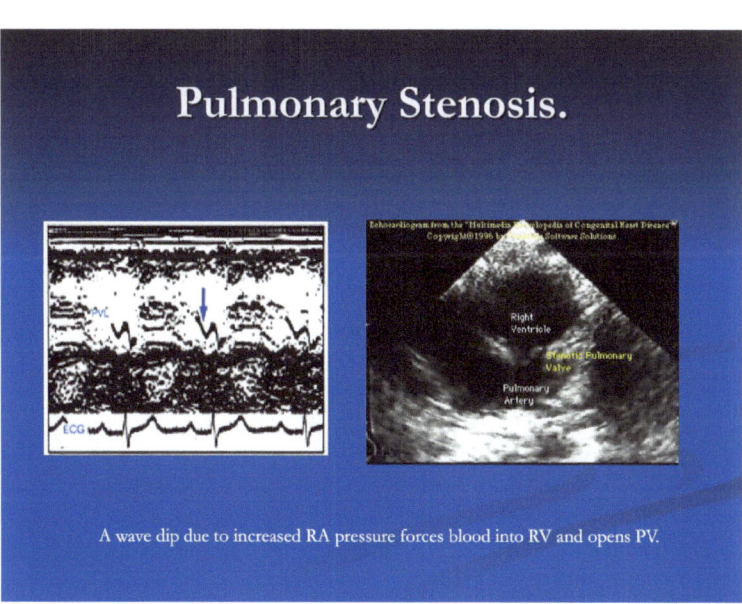

A wave dip due to increased RA pressure forces blood into RV and opens PV.

Pulmonary Stenosis.

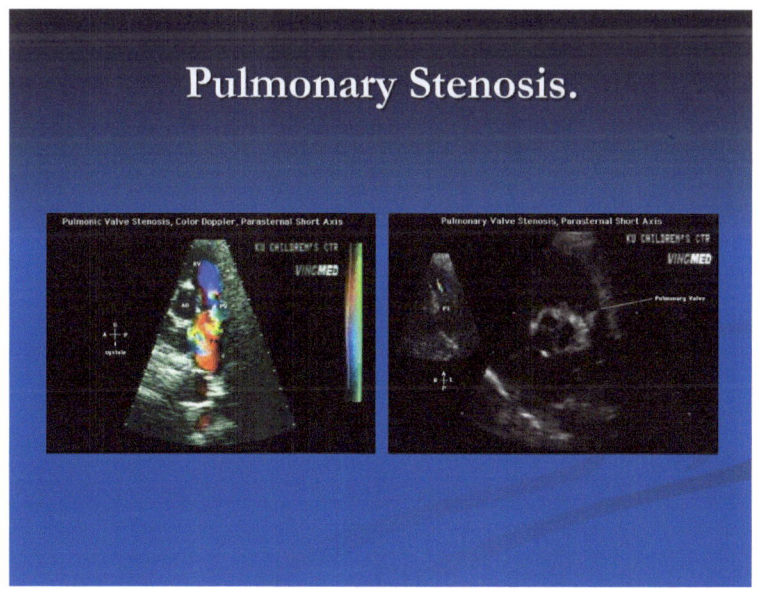

Pulmonary Regurgitation.

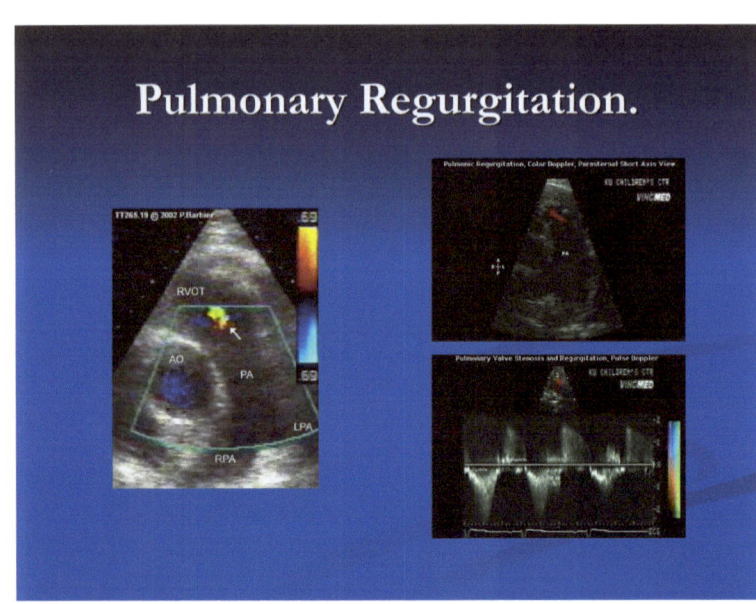

Pulmonary Regurgitation Treated with Prosthetic Pulmonary Valve.

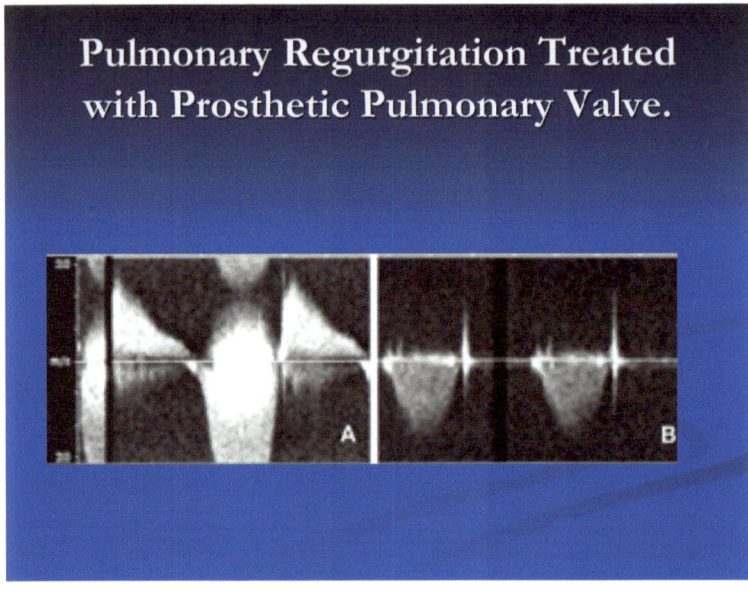

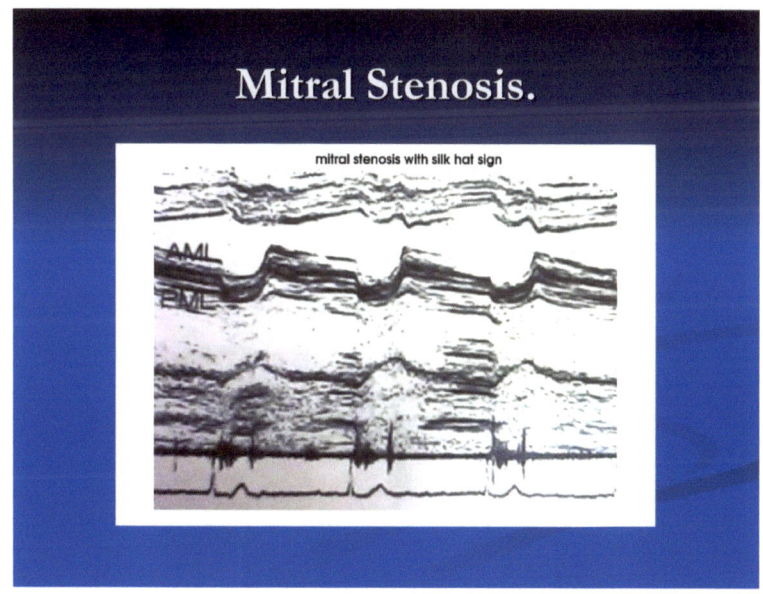

Mitral Stenosis.

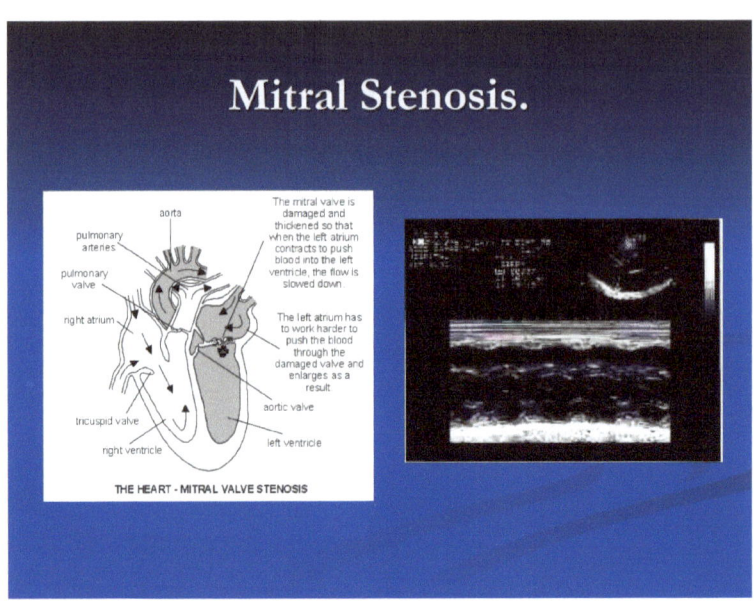

Mitral Stenosis.

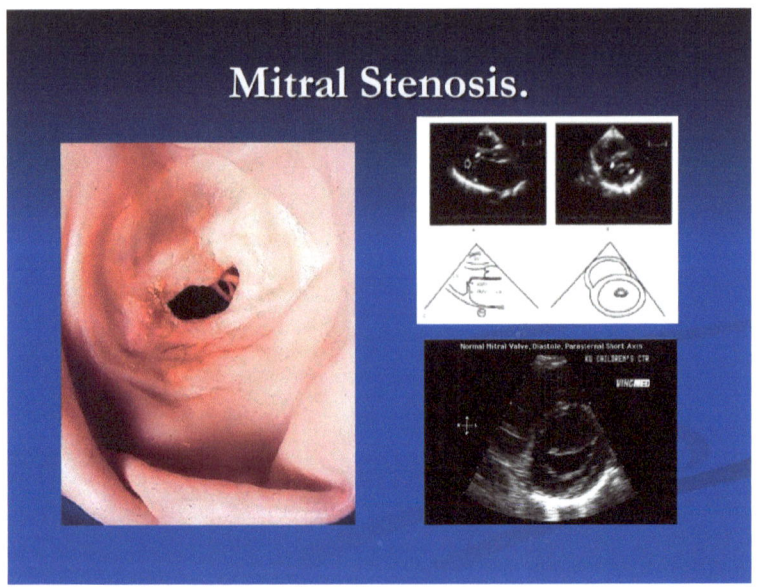

Mitral Valve Area (MVA)

- MVA by Pressure half-time =
  - 1) PV (E point=129 cm/s) = (4)(1.29^2)=6.66 mm Hg.
    - P-1/2= ½ (129) x (0.7") = 90.3 mm Hg
    - P-1/2 time is time to 90.3 mm Hg
  - 2) MVA = 220/(P-1/2t) = eg. 220/181 msec = 1.22 cm^2
- Or
- MVA by DT (deceleration time-time from E point to baseline) =
  - 759/DT = 759/610 msec = 1.24 cm^2
- The shorter the Pressure 1/2, the bigger the valve.
- The shorter the DT, the bigger the valve.
- This means the sharper the drop from E to baseline, the larger the valve.

* 1/1.414 (sq root of 2) = 0.7
P ½ = PHT = pressure half time.

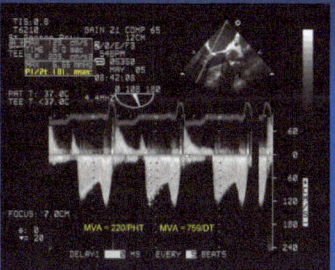

Severity of Mitral Stenosis
Mild = mean gradient < 6 mm Hg and > 1.5 cm^2
Moderate = mean grad 6-16 mm Hg & 1-1.5 cm^2
Severe = mean gradient > 16 mm Hg & < 1 cm^2

Mitral Stenosis.

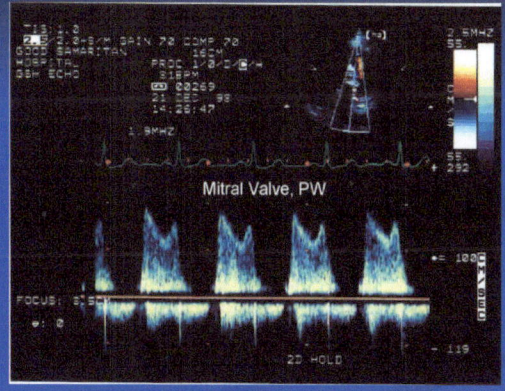

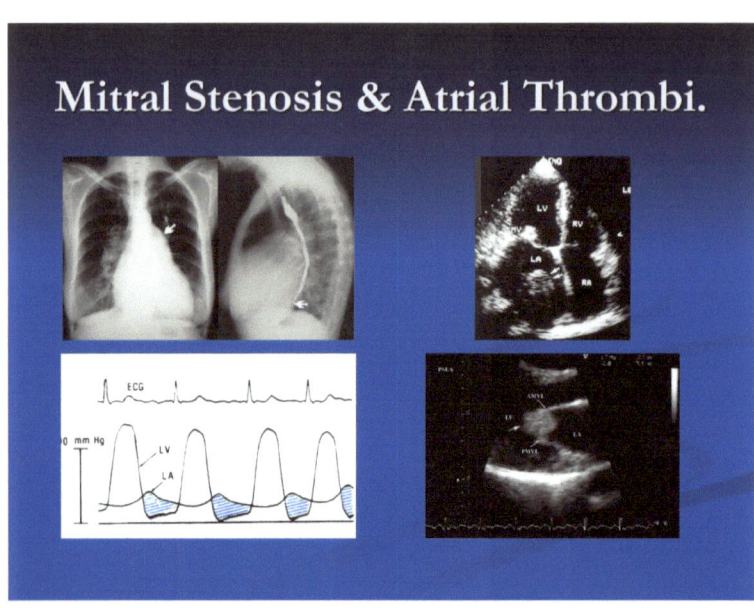

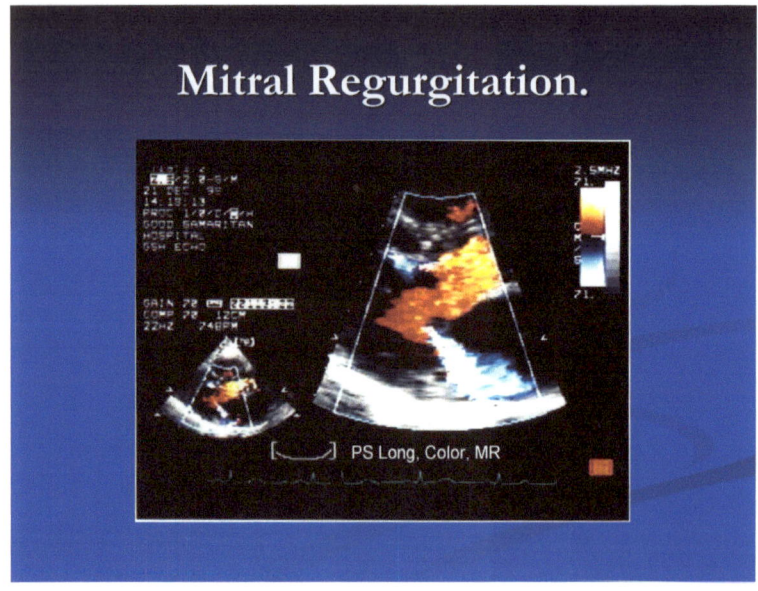

Mitral Regurgitation on Color Flow.

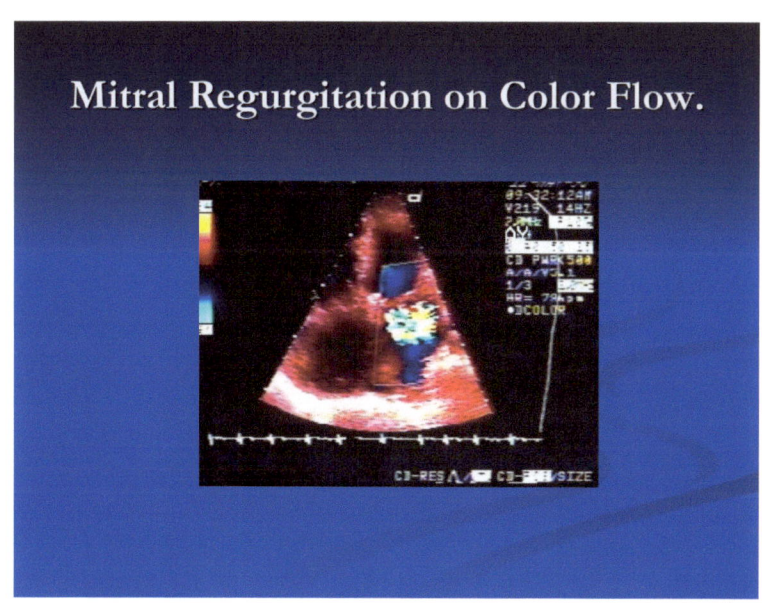

Mitral Regurgitation

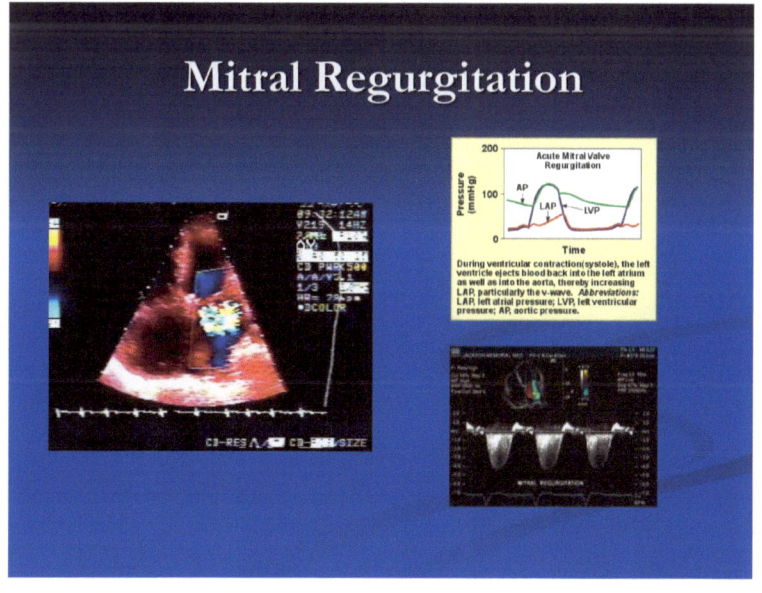

Mitral Valve Prolapse.

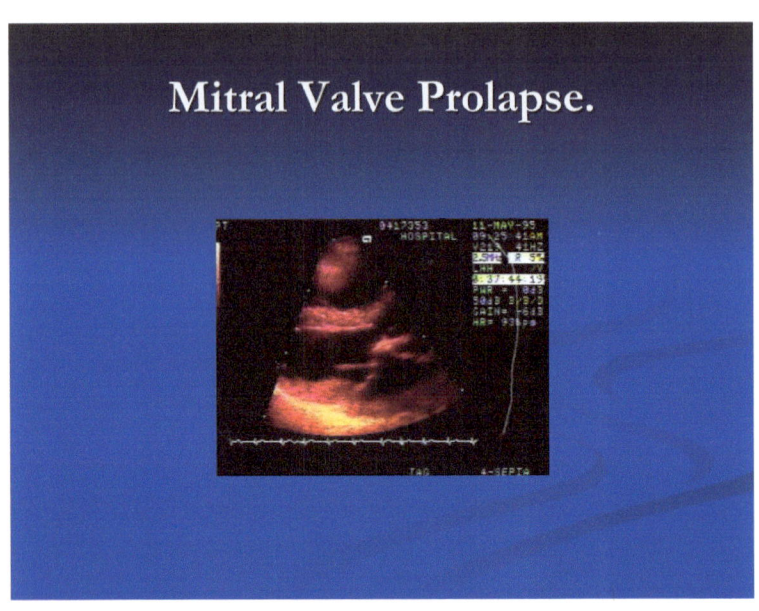

Ventricular Septal Defect.

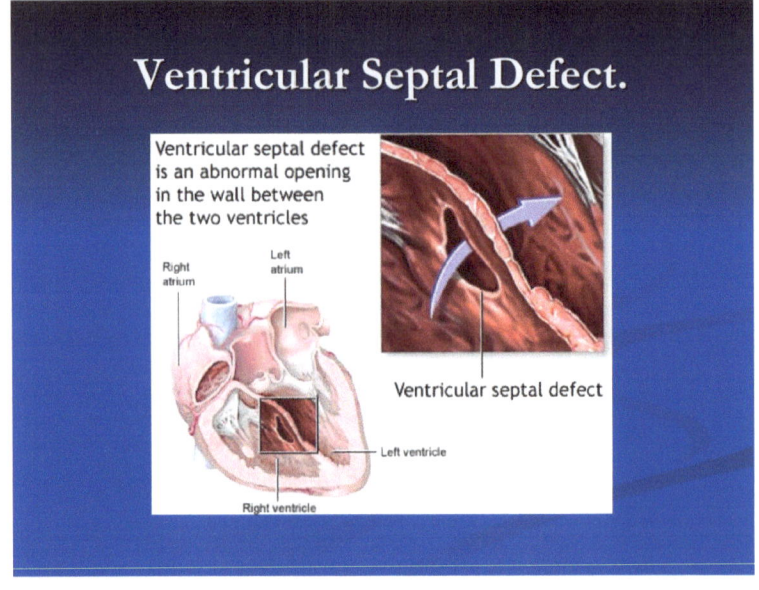

VSD Gradient.

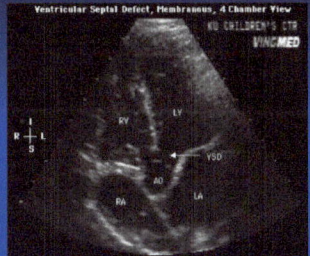
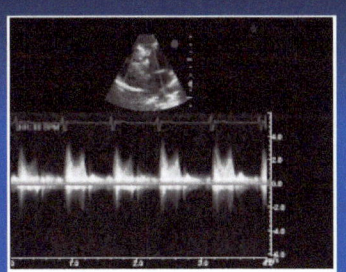

Fig. 3. Continuous-wave Doppler signal across ventricular septal defect. Note the typical M-shaped spectrum with higher peak velocities in early and late systole (zoomed picture on the right side with a peak early systolic velocity of 4 m/s).

VSD gradient = $4V^2$
VSD gradient = $4(4m/s)^2$ = 64 mm Hg
LV peak systolic pressure = sBP (BP cuff) + AoV gradient (PV) if AS present (later in talk).
 Eg. If sBP is 118, AoV PV is 27, then
 LV peak systolic pressure = 118 + 27 = 145 mm Hg.
RV peak systolic pressure = LVESP − VSD gradient = 145 − 64 = 81 mm Hg
 Similar to RVSP calculated with TR.

Aortic Stenosis.

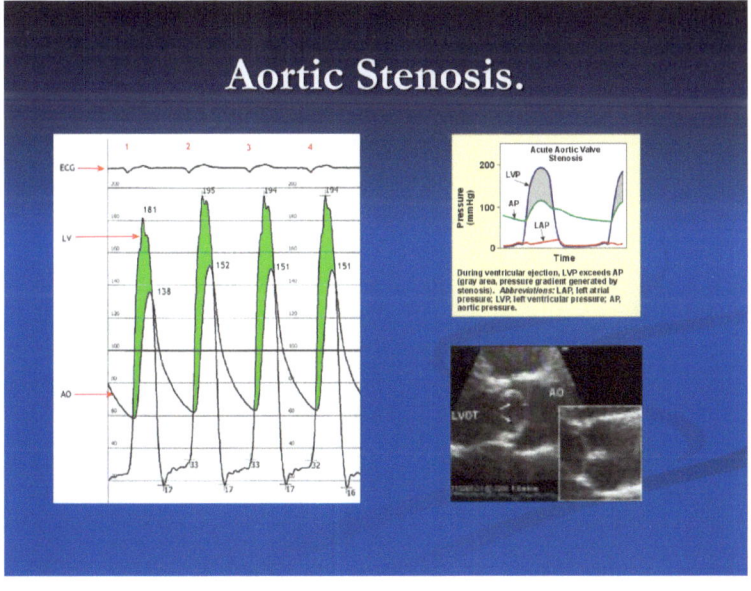

Gradient Across AoV in Patient with BP of 132/80 mm Hg.

- Peak Aortic Valve Gradient = $(4V^2)$
- Velocity (V) by doppler is 3 meters/second.
- $PV^* = (4)(3^2) = 36$ mm Hg
- Peak systolic LV pressure = 132 (sBP) + 36 (gradient pressure) = 168 mm Hg.
- This person has "Mild" AS.

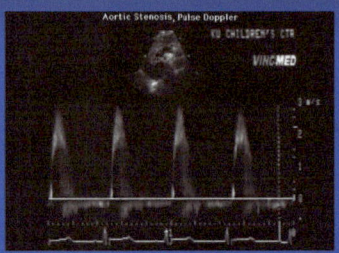

- PV gradient across AoV
- 16-36 mm Hg = Mild AS
- 36-80 mm Hg = Moderate AS
- > 80 mm Hg = Severe AS

Velocity Time Integral

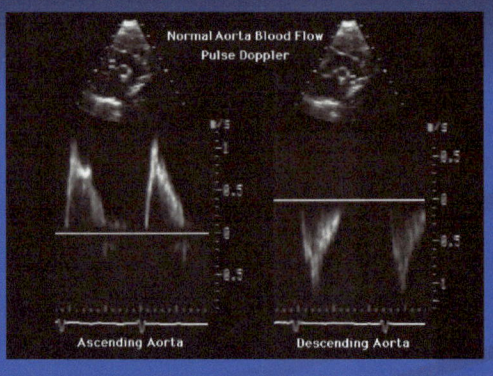

Aortic Valve Area by VTI

- VTI (velocity time integral) = the Stroke Distance (cm)
  - Measured by doppler (area under the curve)
- CSA (cross sectional area) = cm^2 =
  - Πr^2
  - Or $(0.785)(diameter^2)$
- Stroke Volume (cm^3) = Blood Flow (Q) =
  - CSA x VTI = $(0.785)(diameter^2)$ x VTI
- Aortic Valve Area Continuity Equation =
  - CSA_{LVOT} x VTI_{LVOT} = CSA_{AV} x VTI_{AV}
  - $CSA_{AV} = \frac{(0.785)(LVOT\ diameter^2)(VTI_{LVOT})}{VTI_{AV}}$

AoV Area by VTI

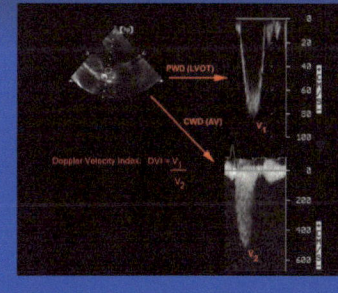
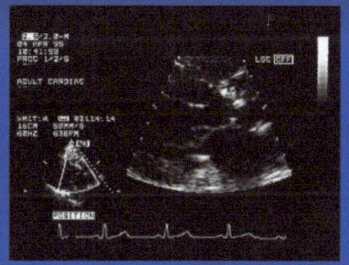

Aortic and Mitral Stenosis (RHD).

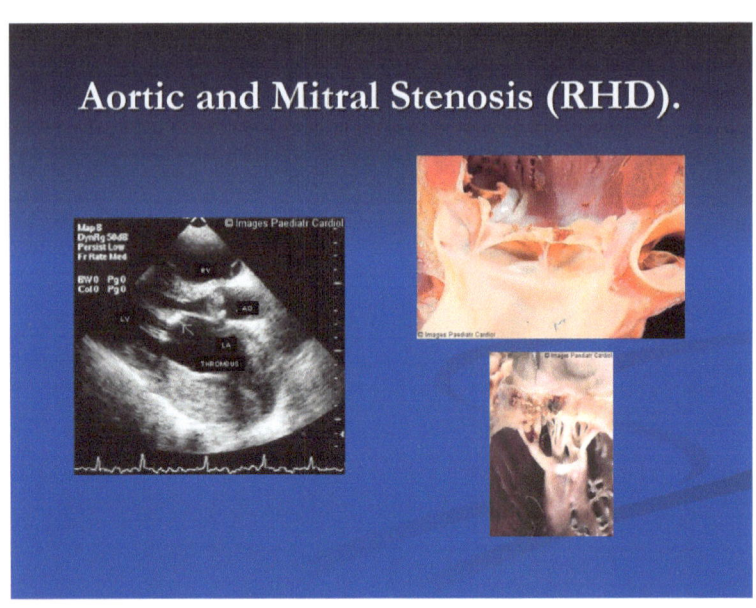

Aortic Regurgitation.

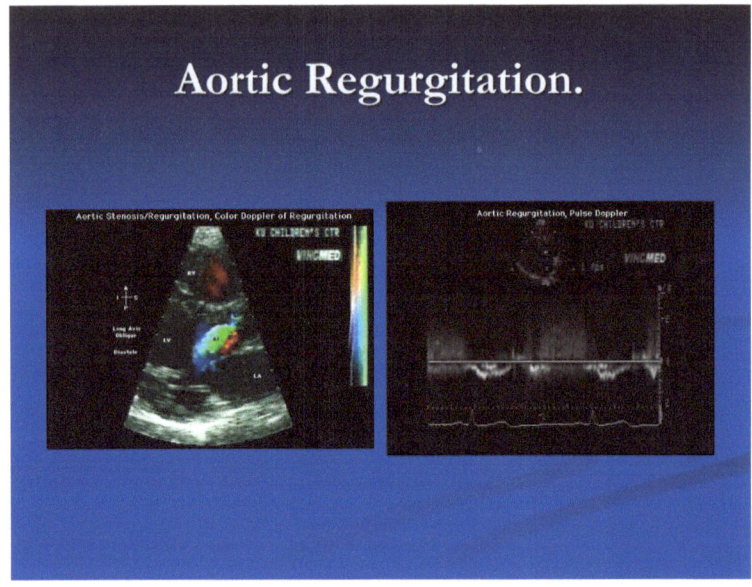

AI Velocity Decay Slope.

- The more gradual the decline (slope) the milder the AI. The more rapid the drop, the greater the AI.
- Two methods to measure AI.
  - 1) DT (deceleration time)
    - Steeper slope (worse AI) equals shorter DT.
    - In this example is 240 cm/sec.
  - 2) PHT measured on screen.
    - Steeper slope (worse AI) equals smaller PHT.
    - In this example is 442 msec.

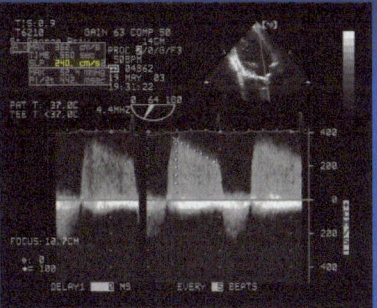

Classification of Aortic Regurgitation:
Mild = DT < 2.0 m/sec and PHT > 550 msec
Moderate = DT 2.0-3.5 m/sec and PHT 550-300 msec
Severe = DT > 3.5 m/sec and PHT < 300 msec. Also diastolic VTI in descending aorta > 15 cm.

AI by Color Flow Doppler.

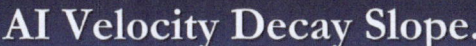

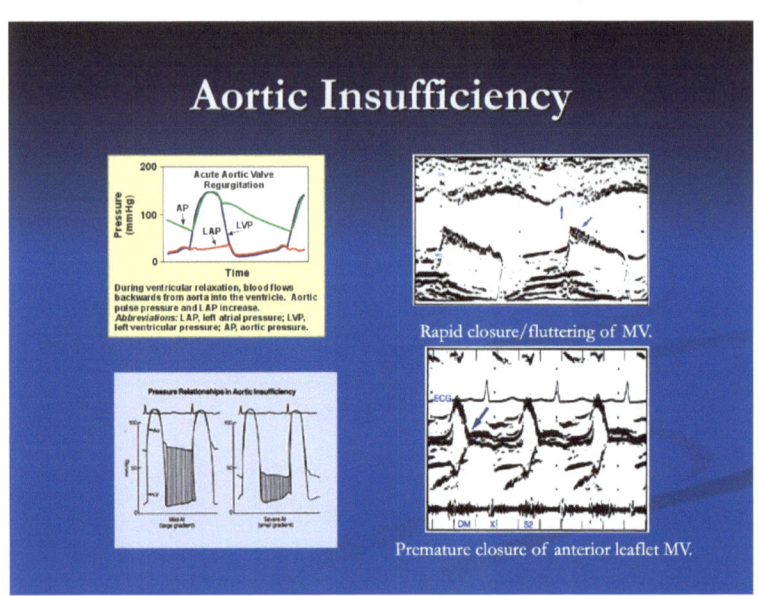
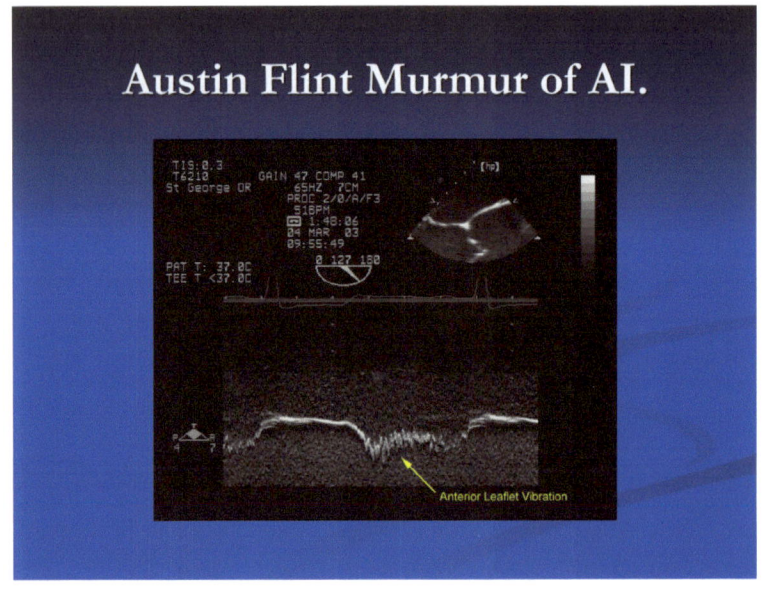

Idiopathic Hypertrophic Sub-aortic Stenosis.

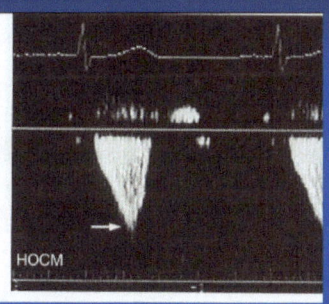
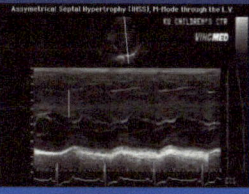
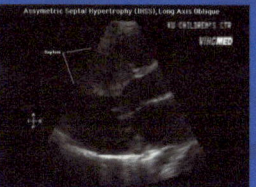

Subaortic Membrane

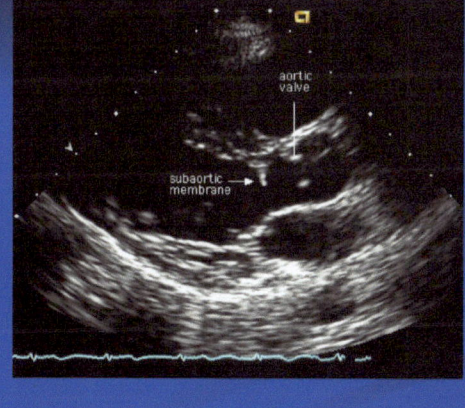

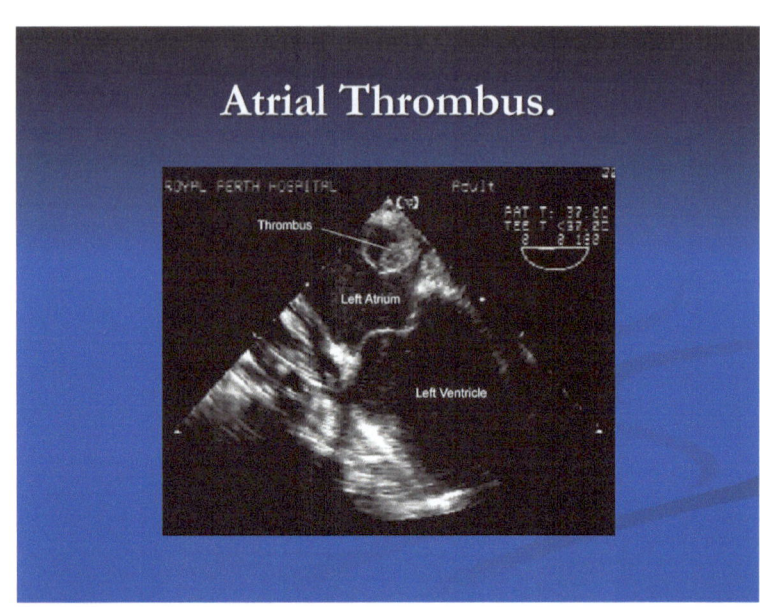

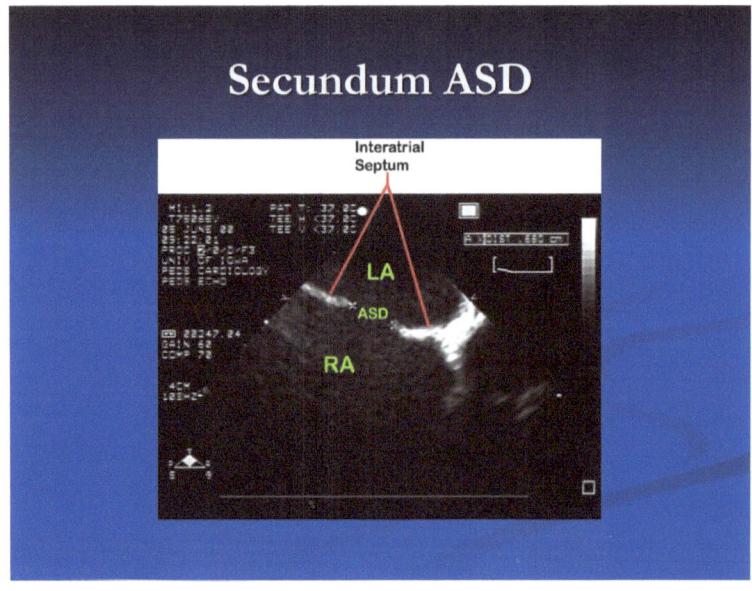

Color Flow Through ASD

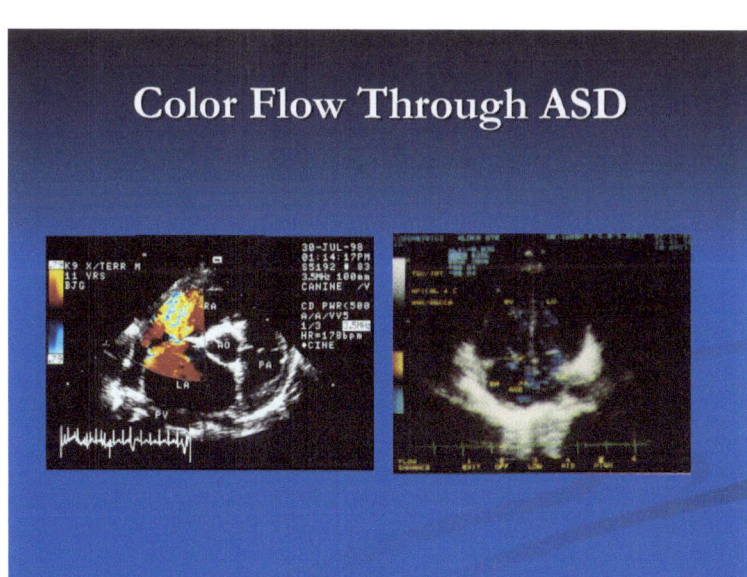

Primary Cardiac Lymphoma

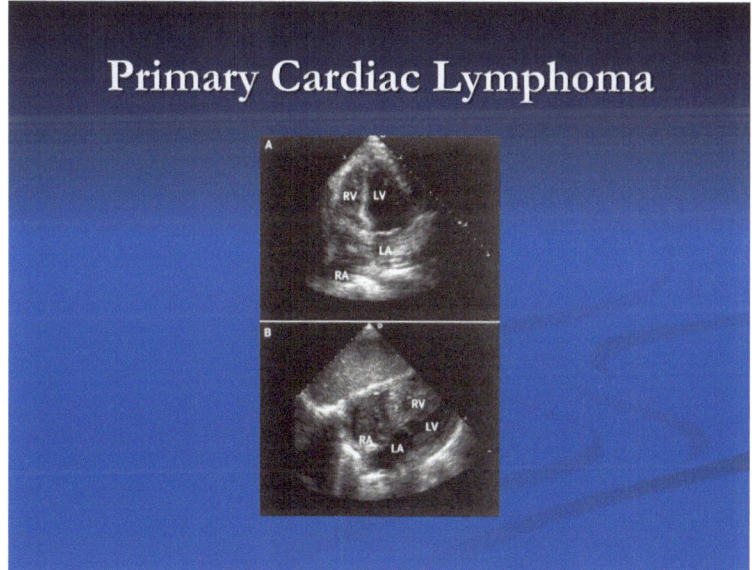

Cardiac Tamponade

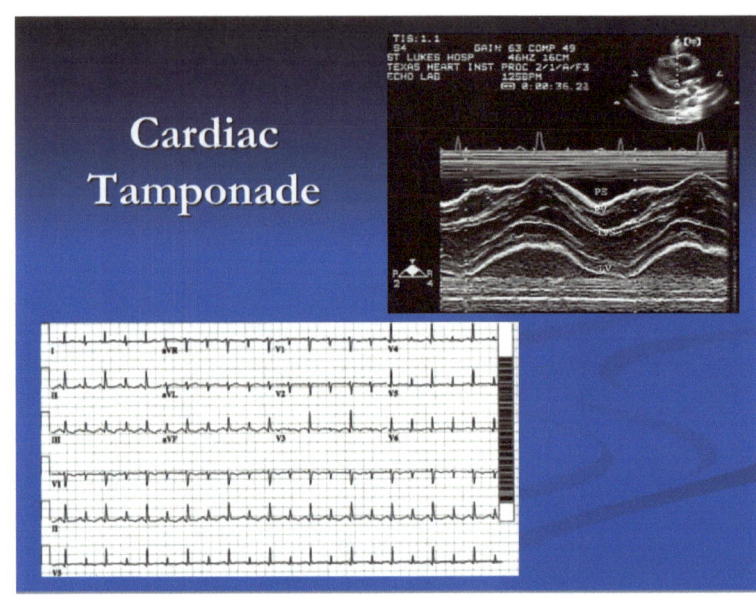

Pericardial Tamponade

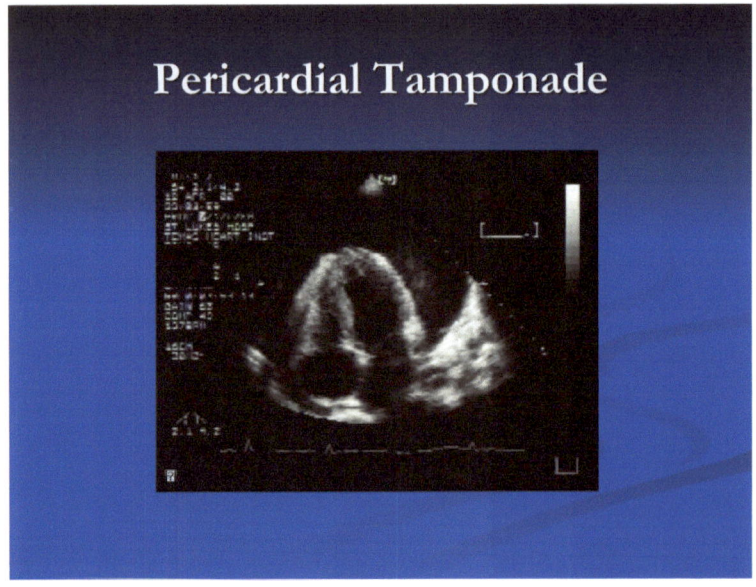

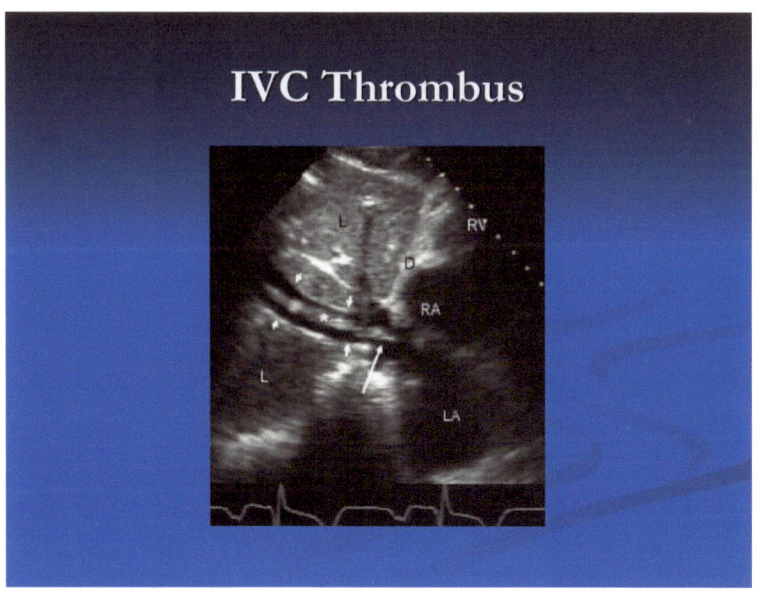

The ability to read and interpret Cardiac Echos provides an extremely useful tool in the care and management of patients. This series of slides developed by myself for the training of physicians and students provides the foundation upon which to build your understanding, care and management of patients using Echocardiography.

www.ingramcontent.com/pod-product-compliance
Lightning Source LLC
Chambersburg PA
CBHW041943240526
45473CB00033B/491